THE COMPLETE NOOM DIET COOKBOOK

A quick and easy, delicious and healthy recipes for Sustainable Weight Loss and Healthy Living

by

Mary Cynthia

Copyright (c)

Table of Contents

INTRODUCTION

Welcome to "The Complete Noom Diet Cookbook" your go-to resource for preparing scrumptious and wholesome meals that follow the Noom Diet's tenets. Regardless of your level of experience with Noom or where you are on your road to healthy living, this cookbook is meant to help you make thoughtful food decisions without compromising taste.

Overview of the Noom Diet
We give a thorough introduction to the Noom Diet in the first segment, going

over its main ideas and tenets. Discover how Noom's color-coded food classification system works to help you make well-informed food decisions based on nutritional density.

Tips for a Successful Noom Diet:
Starting a new diet regimen may be

thrilling as well as difficult. We provide

helpful hints and techniques in this part

to ensure your success with the Noom

Diet. These tips, which cover everything

from grocery shopping to mindful

eating, are designed to make your Noom

experience successful, joyful, and long-

lasting.

Prepare yourself for a tasty journey supporting your fitness and health objectives. "The Complete Noom Diet Cookbook" is your companion in adopting a lifestyle that feeds your body and mind, not merely a compilation of recipes. Let's enjoy the ride together.

CHAPTER 1

Healthy Start Smoothie Bowl

Ingredients:

Regarding the Smoothie:
- One frozen banana, cut

- A half-cup of frozen berry mixture (raspberries, blueberries, and strawberries)

- half a cup of spinach leaves

- half a cup of Greek yogurt

- Half a cup of almond milk

- One spoonful of chia seeds

Add-ons:

- One-fourth cup granola (minimal sugar)

- One tablespoon of shredded coconut without sugar

- Fresh berries

- One tablespoon of honey

Get the Smoothie Base Ready

Blend together the frozen banana, spinach, Greek yogurt, almond milk, mixed berries, and chia seeds using a blender.

Blend till creamy and smooth. To get the right consistency, thin out any excess mixture by adding a small amount of almond milk.

Put the Bowl Together:

Transfer the smoothie into a bowl, making sure the top is uniformly smooth.

Include toppings:

To add more crunch and texture to the smoothie base, evenly sprinkle the granola on top.

For a touch of the tropics, sprinkle the unsweetened shredded coconut on top.

Offer some fresh berries as a garnish to offer some color and extra nutrients.

Drizzle Optional:

Dust the toppings with a spoonful of honey if you're feeling particularly decadent. To adhere to the Noom Diet's tenets, always remember to consume it in moderation.

Savor It with Mindfulness:

Enjoy the vivid hues and textures of your Healthy Start Smoothie Bowl for a moment.

Savor the tastes and nurture your body with healthful nutrients while you attentively enjoy every bite.

Veggie-packed Omelette

Ingredients:

- Two big eggs

- Diced bell peppers, a quarter cup (assorted colors)

- one-fourth cup of chopped tomatoes

- one-fourth cup of red onion, chopped

- one-fourth cup finely chopped spinach

- one-fourth cup of sliced mushrooms

- One tablespoon of olive oil

- To taste, add salt and pepper.
- Fresh herbs for garnish, such parsley or chives

Get the veggies ready:

In a nonstick skillet, warm the olive oil over medium heat.

To the skillet, add the diced bell peppers, tomatoes, red onion, spinach, and mushrooms. Sauté the vegetables for three to five minutes, or until they are soft.

Beat the Eggs:

Beat the eggs until they are well-beaten in a bowl. Add a dash of pepper and salt for seasoning.

Pour Eggs Over Vegetables:

Over the skillet with sautéed vegetables, pour the beaten eggs. Let the eggs settle on top of the veggies.

Prepare the Omelette:

Using a spatula to lift the edges, cook the omelet over medium heat, allowing the raw eggs to run below. Continue until the tops of the eggs are slightly runny but the insides are mostly set.

Fold and Finish:

Using a spatula, delicately fold the omelet in half after the eggs are mostly set.

Cook for a further one to two minutes, or until the veggies are soft and the eggs are cooked through.

Serve and garnish:

Transfer the omelette to a platter and top it with freshly chopped herbs.

For a well-balanced dinner, serve it hot and think about combining it with a small dish of fruit or a side of whole-grain toast.

Savor It with Mindfulness:

Enjoy the flavors and colors of your veggie-packed omelette for a bit. Take time to taste each piece slowly and savor the harmony of eggs and nutrient-dense veggies.

Whole Grain Pancakes with Berry Compote

Ingredients:

- Regarding the Pancakes:

- One cup of flour whole wheat

- One spoonful of sugar (or preferred sweetener)

- One-spoonful baking powder

- half a teaspoon of baking soda

- One-fourth teaspoon of salt

- One cup of buttermilk (or yogurt combined with milk)

- One big egg

- Two teaspoons of melted butter

- One teaspoon of vanilla essence

Regarding the Berry Compote:

One cup of mixed berries (strawberries, blueberries, raspberries)

Two teaspoons of pure maple syrup

One tablespoon of lemon juice

Half a teaspoon of extract from vanilla

Instructions
Regarding the Pancakes:

Get the dry ingredients ready.

Mix the whole wheat flour, sugar, baking soda, baking powder, and salt in a sizable bowl.

Blend the Wet Substances:

Mix the melted butter, egg, buttermilk, and vanilla extract in a separate basin.

Integrate the dry and wet ingredients:

Mixing until just mixed, pour the wet components into the dry ingredients. It's alright to have some lumps; don't over mix.

Prepare the Pancakes:

Over medium heat, preheat a nonstick skillet or griddle. Use cooking spray or a tiny bit of butter to grease.

Pour 1/4 cup of batter for each pancake onto the griddle. Fry until surface bubbles appear, then turn and continue cooking until both sides are golden brown.

Keep Warm:

While you make the berry compote, keep the pancakes warm on a platter covered with a fresh kitchen towel.

Regarding the Berry Compote:

Get the berries ready:

Put the mixed berries, lemon juice, and maple syrup in a saucepan.

Simmer:

Over medium heat, bring the mixture to a moderate simmer. Simmer for five to seven minutes or until the syrup thickens and the berries become tender.

Include Vanilla:

After taking the compote off the stove, mix in the vanilla essence.

Serve:

Put the Pancakes Together:

Spoon plenty of the warm berry compote over the top of the stacked whole-grain pancakes.

Savor It with Mindfulness:

Take your time and enjoy the delicious burst of flavors from the berry compote in every bite of these whole-grain pancakes.

CHAPTER 2

Quinoa and Chickpea Salad

Ingredients:

Regarding the Salad:

One cup of washed and cooked quinoa, following the directions on the package

One can of washed and drained chickpeas

one cup of diced cucumbers

One cup of cherry tomatoes, halved

Half a cup of diced red bell pepper

One-fourth cup of finely chopped red onion

One-fourth cup of fresh parsley

Instructions:

Regarding the Salad:

1. Prepare Quinoa: After giving it a quick rinse in cold water, prepare it as directed on the packaging. After cooking, use a fork to fluff it up and allow it to cool to room temperature.

2. Cook Vegetables: Cooked quinoa, chickpeas, cucumber, cherry tomatoes, red bell pepper, red onion, and fresh

parsley should all be combined in a big mixing dish.

Serve:

1. Plate and Portion: Transfer the Quinoa and Chickpea Salad onto a sizable serving bowl or place it onto individual plates.

2. Garnish (Optional): For a pop of color, garnish with extra fresh parsley.

3. Savor It with Mindfulness: Enjoy the variety of flavors and textures in this healthy salad that is loaded with nutrition from chickpeas and quinoa.

Not only is quinoa and chickpea salad filling, but it's also a healthy, light dinner that's ideal for people on the Noom Diet.

Grilled Chicken and Veggie Wrap

Ingredients:

Regarding the Chicken Grilled:

Two skinless and boneless chicken breasts

One tablespoon of olive oil

One teaspoon of dehydrated oregano

One teaspoon of powdered garlic

To taste, add salt and pepper.

Regarding the Veggie Filling:

One cup of thinly sliced bell peppers (assorted colors)

One cup of thinly sliced zucchini

Half a cup of cherry tomatoes

One tablespoon of olive oil

To taste, add salt and pepper.

For the Wrap:

Four tortillas, whole-grain or spinach

One cup of freshly cleaned spinach
leaves

Half a cup of crumbled feta cheese
(optional)

Tzatziki sauce or Greek yogurt for
serving

Instructions:

Regarding the Chicken Grilled:

(1) Grill or Pan Prep: Turn the heat up to
medium-high on your grill or grill pan.

(2) To season chicken, combine olive oil, garlic powder, dried oregano, salt, and pepper in a bowl. Apply this mixture to the chicken breasts.

(3) Grill Chicken: Grill the chicken breasts until they are 165°F (74°C) on the inside, 6 to 8 minutes per side. Before slicing, let them a few minutes to rest.

Regarding the Veggie Filling:

(1) Sauté Vegetables: Heat some olive oil in a skillet over medium heat. Add the

cherry tomatoes, zucchini, and chopped
bell peppers. Add pepper and salt for
seasoning. Sauté the vegetables for 5 to 7
minutes, or until they are crisp-tender.

(2) Mix with Chicken: In a skillet,
combine the sautéed vegetables and the
grilled chicken slices. Toss until
thoroughly mixed.

The Noom Diet is a fantastic fit for
people who follow the Grilled Chicken
and Veggie Wrap because it's a
delicious, well-balanced meal that offers
a satisfying blend of protein, fiber, and
nutrients.

Lentil and Vegetable Soup

Ingredients:

One cup of dried, rinsed, and drained green or brown lentils

One tablespoon of olive oil

One diced onion

Two diced and peeled carrots

Two diced celery stalks

Three minced garlic cloves

One teaspoon of cumin powder

One teaspoon of finely ground coriander

One teaspoon of smoky paprika

One bay leaf

Six cups of vegetable stock

One 14-oz can have chopped, undrained tomatoes

Two cups of chopped kale or spinach

Add salt and pepper to taste.

Chopped fresh parsley (for garnish)

(1) Prepare the lentils by giving them a quick rinse in cold water and putting them aside.

(2) Sauté Vegetables: Place a large saucepan over medium heat with olive oil. Add the celery, carrots, and diced onion. Sauté the veggies for five to seven minutes, or until they become tender.

(3) Add Garlic and Spices: Toss in the minced garlic, bay leaf, smoked paprika, ground cumin, and ground coriander. Add the spices and sauté for a further one to two minutes, or until aromatic.

(4) Combine Lentils and Broth: Fill the saucepan with the diced tomatoes (including juice), vegetable broth, and washed lentils. Mix thoroughly to blend.

(5) Simmer: After bringing the soup to a boil, turn down the heat. The lentils should be soft after 25 to 30 minutes of simmering under cover.

(6) Add Leafy Greens: Cook for a further five minutes, or until the greens have wilted, after stirring in the chopped spinach or kale.

(7) Add salt and pepper to taste while seasoning the soup. Take out the bay leaf. Add freshly cut parsley as a garnish.

(8) Pour the Lentil and Vegetable Soup into bowls and serve warm. Warm-up and savor.

(9) Savor It with Mindfulness: This cozy soup is a substantial and nutritious blend of lentils, veggies, and aromatic spices.

In addition to being a filling and healthful supper, lentil and vegetable soup also adhere to the Noom Diet's tenets by offering a healthy proportion of fiber, protein, and other vital elements.

CHAPTER 3

Baked Salmon with Lemon-Dill Sauce

Ingredients:

Four salmon fillets, skin-on or skinless, approximately 6 ounces each

Two teaspoons of olive oil

One teaspoon of powdered garlic

One teaspoon of powdered onion

One teaspoon of dried dill

To taste, add salt and pepper.

Slices of lemon (for garnish)

Regarding the Lemon-Dill Sauce:

Half a cup of plain, fat-free Greek yogurt

Two tablespoons of freshly chopped dill

One tablespoon of lemon juice

One teaspoon of Dijon mustard

To taste, add salt and pepper.

Instructions:

Regarding the Baked Salmon:

(1) Set the oven's temperature to 400°F or 200°C.

(2) To prepare the salmon, pat dry with a paper towels the fillets. Place the salmon fillets, skin-side down, on a lightly oiled surface if using skin-on salmon.

(3) To season salmon, combine olive oil, dried dill, onion and garlic powders, salt, and pepper in a small bowl. Make sure the salmon fillets are evenly coated by brushing them with the mixture.

(4) Bake the salmon for 12 to 15 minutes, or until it is cooked through

and flake readily with a fork, in an oven that has been warmed.

(5) Before serving, sprinkle some lemon slices on top of the baked salmon.

Regarding the Lemon-Dill Sauce:

(1) Combine Greek yogurt, lemon juice, Dijon mustard, chopped fresh dill, salt, and pepper in a small bowl.

(2) A spoonful of Lemon-Dill Sauce can be served on the side or top of the baked salmon.

(3) Enjoy the zesty zing of the Lemon-Dill Sauce with the luscious and delicious Baked Salmon. Savor it over a

bed of steamed vegetables or your preferred side dishes.

Vegetarian Stir-Fry with Brown Rice

Ingredients:

Two cups of brown rice, cooked

Two teaspoons of sesame oil

One 14-oz block of extra-firm, pressed and diced tofu

One cup florets of broccoli

One thinly sliced bell pepper in a variety of colors

One carrot, thinly sliced

One cup of blanched snap peas

One cup of sliced mushrooms

Three minced garlic cloves

One tablespoon of grated ginger

Two teaspoons of soy sauce (low sodium)

One teaspoon of hoisin sauce

one tablespoon of rice vinegar

One teaspoon of sesame seeds, as a garnish

Sliced green onions (for garnish)

Instructions:

(1) After pressing the tofu to get rid of extra water, chop it into bite-sized pieces.

(2) Follow the cooking directions on the package for brown rice. Put aside.

(3) Sesame oil should be heated over medium-high heat in a sizable wok or skillet. Stir-fry the cubed tofu until it turns golden and begins to crisp up. Take out the tofu and place it aside.

(4) If necessary, add a little extra sesame oil to the same wok. Fry the ginger and garlic until aromatic.

Add the snap peas, carrot, bell pepper, broccoli, and mushrooms. Sauté the veggies for five to seven minutes, or until they are crisp-tender.

(5) Add the cooked tofu and the sautéed vegetables back to the wok. Combine by tossing everything together.

(6) Mix the rice vinegar, hoisin sauce, and soy sauce in a small basin. Mix thoroughly after adding the sauce to the stir-fry.

(7) To the wok, add the cooked brown rice. Stir-fry for a further two to three minutes, or until well cooked and mixed.

(8) Add some sesame seeds and sliced green onions to the vegetarian stir-fry as garnish.

(9) Warm up the Vegetarian Stir-Fry with Brown Rice and enjoy the delicious blend of tastes and textures.

CHAPTER 4

Guilt-Free Guacamole

Ingredients:

Two ripe avocados, seeded and de-seeded

One chopped tomato

A quarter of a cup of coarsely chopped red onion

One minced garlic clove

One juiced lime

Two tablespoons of freshly cut cilantro

To taste, add salt and pepper.

Instructions:

(1) Mash the ripe avocados with a fork in a bowl.

(2) To the mashed avocados, add diced tomato, chopped red onion, minced garlic, lime juice, and chopped cilantro. Blend thoroughly.

(3) To taste, add salt and pepper for seasoning. As needed, adjust the seasoning and lime juice.

(4) (Optional) Before serving, the guacamole should be chilled for at least half an hour to bring out the flavors.

(5) Serve the guilt-free guacamole as a tasty garnish for salads and main meals, or with whole-grain tortilla chips.

Greek Yogurt and Berry Parfait

Ingredients:

1 cup plain, fat-free Greek yogurt

One cup of mixed berries, including raspberries, blueberries, and strawberries

A quarter of a cup of low-sugar granola

One spoonful of honey (to be used for drizzling)

Instructions:

(1) Start with a layer of Greek yogurt in a glass or bowl.

(2) Spread some mixed berries over the yogurt.

(3) Over the berries, scatter some low-sugar granola.

(4) Continue layering until you reach the top of the bowl or glass, and then add a final layer of berries.

(5) (Optional) If desired, drizzle some honey over the top for further sweetness.

(6) This is a tasty and healthy Greek Yogurt and Berry Parfait. Savor it as a filling dessert or a nutritious breakfast.

Spiced Roasted Chickpeas

Ingredients:

Two cans (15 oz. each) of rinsed and drained chickpeas

Two tablespoons of olive oil

One teaspoon of cumin powder

One teaspoon of smoky paprika

Half a teaspoon of powdered garlic

Half a teaspoon of powdered onion

One-fourth teaspoon of cayenne (adjust according to taste)

Add salt to taste.

Instructions:

(1) Set oven temperature to 400°F or 200°C.

(2) Using a paper towel, pat the drained chickpeas dry to eliminate any remaining moisture.

(3) Chickpeas should be combined with olive oil, salt, cayenne pepper, onion powder, smoked paprika, ground cumin, and garlic powder in a bowl. Make careful to coat the chickpeas thoroughly.

(4) Arrange the seasoned chickpeas on a baking pan in a single layer. Roast, shaking the pan halfway through, for 25 to 30 minutes, or until brown and crispy in the preheated oven.

(5) Before serving, lct the roasted chickpeas with spice settle.

(6) These Spiced Roasted Chickpeas make a tasty and crunchy snack. They are also delicious added to salads or used as a soup topper.

CHAPTER 5

WEEK 1:

First Day:

Healthy Start Smoothie Bowl for breakfast

Quinoa and Chickpea Salad for lunch

Lemon-Dill Sauced Baked Salmon for Dinner

Snack: Veggie sticks with guilt-free guacamole

Berry compote and whole grain pancakes for breakfast

Lunch would be brown rice and a vegetarian stir-fry.

Lentils and veggies soup for dinner

Berries and Greek Yogurt Parfait for snack

Omelette with veggies for breakfast

Mixed greens and spiced roasted chickpeas for Lunch.

Veggie wrap with grilled chicken for dinner

Fruits (Apples, berries)

Greek yogurt, granola, and sliced banana for breakfast

Quinoa and Chickpea Salad for lunch

Tomato and basil sauce over spaghetti squash for dinner

Walnuts or almonds for a snack

Chia seeds overnight oats topped with mixed berries for Breakfast

Lentil and vegetable soup for lunch

Sweet potato skillet with turkey for dinner.

Carrot hummus for snack

Avocado Toast with Poached Egg for Breakfast

Grilled chicken or a Greek salad with tofu for Lunch.

Brown rice stir-fried with vegetables for dinner.

Pineapple-flavored cottage cheese for snack.

Mango, banana, and spinach blended into a green smoothie for breakfast

Quinoa and black bean bowl for lunch

Mediterranean Salsa and Baked Cod for dinner.

Unsalted Mixed Nuts for snack.

First Day:

Berry parfait and Greek yogurt for breakfast

Quinoa salad with grilled chicken for lunch

Enchiladas with sweet potatoes and black beans for dinner

Roasted Chickpeas with Spices for snack

Second Day:

Sliced apple and whole grain pancakes with almond butter for breakfast

Hummus and a lentil and vegetable wrap for lunch

Mango salsa and baked salmon for dinner

Whole Wheat pita chips with guilt-free guacamole for snack

Egg muffins with spinach and feta for breakfast

Stir-fried Vegetable and Chickpeas for lunch

Black beans and quinoa stuffed bell peppers for dinner

Fruit Salad for snack

Sandwich with avocado and tomato for breakfast

Tofu and Mediterranean quinoa salad for lunch

Quinoa with Shrimp and Vegetable Skewers for dinner

Cottage Cheese and Mixed Berries for snack

Banana Walnut Overnight Oats for breakfast

Teriyaki Tofu and Brown Rice Bowl for lunch

Cauliflower rice and vegetable and turkey kebabs for dinner

Walnuts and Honey with Greek Yogurt for snack

Sixth Day:

Honey-flavored Greek yogurt with walnuts for breakfast

Whole grain baguette and capers salad
for lunch

Primavera spaghetti squash for dinner

Bell pepper strips and hummus for
snack

Seventh Day:

Peanut Butter Banana Wrap for
breakfast

Buddha bowl with quinoa and chickpeas
for lunch

Halloumi and grilled vegetable skewers
for dinner

Trail Mix containing nuts and dried
fruits for snack

CHAPTER 6

As we near the end of "The Complete Noom Diet Cookbook," we sincerely hope you have relished the experience of learning how to make savory, wholesome, and filling foods that follow the guidelines of the Noom Diet. Here are a few closing ideas and pointers to remember while you continue on your journey toward health and well-being.

Think back for a moment on the food you have prepared using this cookbook. Think about the flavors you've eaten, the different dishes you've attempted, and how your perspective on food and nutrition may have changed. Honor your accomplishments, no matter how modest, and recognize the constructive

actions you've taken to lead a healthier
lifestyle.

Remain present during meals as you
continue to practice mindful eating.
Enjoy the social aspects of dining, pay
attention to indications of hunger and
fullness, and savor the flavors and
textures of your food. Developing a
mindful eating style benefits your
general well-being in addition to your
physical health.

I hope your Noom Diet adventure brings
your health and happiness. Good eating
and be well!s